Mindful Maturation

Graceful Aging for Baby Boomers

Table of Contents

Chapter 1. Introduction

In this unique Special Report, we delve into the heartwarming journey of "Mindful Maturation: Graceful Aging for Baby Boomers". Bridging the gap between youth and old age, this report celebrates the wisdom and elegance of aging, drenched in a mélange of engaging anecdotes, thoughtful insights, and empowering concepts. We sprinkle a dash of mindfulness, a zest of positivity, and a hefty dose of inspiration to craft a roadmap for anyone navigating the path of graceful aging. With this report in your hands, you're not merely surviving each day but dancing through the art of living mindfully, making every moment count. It's not a technical analysis, rather an irresistible, joyful guide for that golden chapter of your life. We promise you, by the time you finish reading this paragraph, you'll be imagining the wealth of content that lies within, ready to embark on this enlightening journey vibrant with life's ripened fruits! A toast to your refined yet spirited journey ahead, enriched by wisdom, enriched by experience, and, most of all, enriched by joyful acceptance. Purchase this Special Report today and embark on your journey to Mindful Maturation.

Chapter 2. Embracing the Passage of Time

The adventure that is life manifests itself in changing seasons, evolving chapters, and an undaunted progression of time. Each tick of the clock reminds us that not a single moment can exist again, not in the exact facade it showed us. Thus, understanding, accepting, and embracing this journey of time is imperative for our growth, maturation, and flourishing mental health as we march along on life's path.

2.1. The Spectacle of Change

Nature purveys an illustrious example of how change is a critical denominator in the lifecycle of anything and everything. The luscious green leaves of a tree, at the pinnacle of their vigor, with time transform into a beautiful, golden visual spectacle as autumn descends. Without resistance, they don their golden hues, culminating in a display of crimson and orange that is nothing short of a masterpiece. They submit to the inevitable change, gracing it with acceptance and thus deriving beauty out of it.

As human beings, our journey exhibits a similar cycle. Every moment, every decision, every encounter, we are on a constant trajectory of evolution, molding and shaping ourselves in the forge of life's experiences. Each day, we shed an old version of ourselves and embrace a new one, bolstered with the accumulated knowledge, wisdom, and insights of days passed.

2.2. The Beauty of Patina

Just as an antique, valued for its patina, we should celebrate the signs of age, a testament to our experiences, challenges, victories, and survival. Our wrinkles are the lines on a map, guiding us to the moments that have carved our stories. Each line, each gray hair, and each crow's foot narrates the tales of mirth and tears, of ups and downs, of love and loss.

When we look at ourselves, rather than chasing an elusive, media-set standard of beauty, let's endeavor to see the elegance in our existence. Let's appraise the beauty of our journey, the wisdom we hold, and the resilience in our spirit. Let's take pride in our patina, relishing the gratification of a life well-lived.

2.3. Unshackling from the Past

As we step further along in our journey, it's natural for memories and perhaps unfilled desires to surface. It's the past that sometimes tends to shroud our present, casting shadows that make it challenging to discern the light. Yet, it's also the past that aids in illuminating our path ahead. Cementing life's experiences as learnings rather than longings, we can leverage the understandings for a balanced and joyful present, and a mindful and exciting future. Unshackle the past's chains, for it shouldn't be an anchor but a compass, directing you towards a fulfilling journey ahead.

2.4. Tryst with Time

Time is often depicted as an enemy, a stealthy thief snatching away our youth. But, if viewed from a different lens, it is the most loyal companion, a silent walker by our side, an infallible scribe, recording our lives in the annals of existence. Along with time, we grow, we learn, we build, we destroy, we mend, and most importantly, we incessantly move forward.

When you find yourself in front of the mirror, trace your life with the lines of age, and celebrate the journey that each one represents. Remember, aging is not a curse, but a continuous opportunity for growth, development, and the amalgamation of wisdom. It is the opportunity to distill valuable insights from collected experiences and use them to our advantage.

2.5. Cultivating Mindfulness and Gratitude

Mindfulness is the practice of being present at the moment, and at this specific moment lies our true existence. It helps us streamline our focus on the gift that is 'now,' enabling us to embrace every experience and moment thoroughly. Mindfulness intertwined with gratitude magnifies the beauty of life, making us appreciate each blessing, each achievement, and each new day.

Opening our hearts to gratitude, we fill our souls with positivity, spurring the cycle of happiness and contentment. By being grateful for what we have, we foster an environment of abundance, warding off the creeping negativities borne of worries and unnecessary expectations.

Learning to love the passage of time is an art, a melody composed in the rhythm that matches our heartbeats, reverberating through the symphony of life. Understand that it's a part of our existence. A part that makes us realize the value, beauty, and ephemeral nature of moments and teaches us to live them fully. So, let's sway along, let's age gracefully, let's embrace the passage of time, and let's immerse ourselves in the bliss of mindful maturation.

Chapter 3. Decoding the Secrets of Mindfulness

Mindfulness, at its core, is all about absolute present-moment awareness - the pure, unadulterated focus on the now. Throughout our existence, we inadvertently train our minds to wander, fret about the past and future, rarely being truly 'present'. Mindfulness encourages us to break these chains, to live in the 'here and now'. This allows us to experience life in its truest form—bright, vivid, and pulsating with rich, intricate detail.

3.1. Understanding Mindfulness

Let's consider a simple exercise. Take a pause from this reading and simply observe your surroundings for a minute. Notice the hum of the air conditioner, the smell of the coffee on the table, the texture of the paper beneath your fingers, or perhaps the subtle tension in your shoulders. This focus on the present moment, without judgment or analysis, encapsulates the essence of mindfulness.

When we're mindful, we are, in essence, detaching ourselves from the whirlwind of our thoughts and feelings, observing rather than getting entangled, and thus gaining clarity and peace of mind. It's about training your mind to stay where your body is, truly in the present moment, regardless of what you are doing.

3.2. The Science Behind Mindfulness

Modern research explains that mindful practice can bring about structural and functional alterations in the brain that enhance mental and emotional health. Mindfulness affects the prefrontal cortex - the region responsible for cognitive activities, such as decision making, focus, and awareness. It also has a significant impact on our amygdala, the center for emotions, fear, and stress.

A regular practice of mindfulness strengthens the neural pathways that help foster cognitive flexibility, stress resilience, emotional balance, enhanced focus, and a deep sense of peace. In simpler terms, the more you practice mindfulness, the more mental and emotional strength you cultivate.

3.3. Embedding Mindfulness in Daily Life

Contrary to popular belief, mindfulness is not just for meditation sessions. It can seep into every corner of our daily life—be it eating, walking, listening, or even dishwashing. Mindful eating, for example, is experiencing the texture, smell, taste, and sound of our food. It's about appreciating the journey of the food, from the field to our plate and finally, to each cell of our body.

Similarly, a mindful walk isn't necessarily a long hike amidst untouched natural beauty, but any walk where you consciously observe each step, the alternation of your left and right foot, the soft sinking of your soles on the ground, the sensation of air brushing past your skin, and your body's gentle rhythm as it moves forward.

Such mindful moments seep color and joy into daily life, making mundane tasks enjoyable and our senses sharper and more alive.

3.4. Techniques for Cultivating Mindfulness

While mindfulness can be practiced in every moment, certain specific exercises can help cultivate this ability. Mindful breathing is one such exercise. It involves purely focusing on the sensation of breath, the rise and fall of the abdomen, the coolness of air entering your nostrils, and the subtle pause between the in-breath and out-breath.

'Body scan' is another powerful mindfulness exercise which cultivates an acute awareness of our body. It involves mentally scanning your body from head to toe, observing each muscle, joint, and organ, the pulsations, tensions, and sensations within, fostering a strong mind-body connection.

Practicing these exercises, beginning with short time intervals and gradually increasing the duration, can help you cultivate mindfulness.

3.5. Mindfulness and Aging

As we age, our brains naturally tend to lose some of their cognitive flexibility and memory capacity. However, by practicing mindfulness, we can significantly slow down this process, maintaining cognitive sharpness and mental health as we age. Mindfulness, with its powerful impacts on stress, anxiety, and depression, gifts us a profound inner peace, a space of quiet and solace within ourselves, which indeed is a priceless boon as we navigate through the golden years of our lives.

By integrating mindfulness into your daily routine, you not only transform your perception towards aging but also infuse each day with a dash of joy and serenity. It creates an aging process that's not merely about surviving, but thriving with grace and vitality, completely in tune with the depth and beauty of each passing moment. Your later years then become a time of celebration of experience, wisdom, and mindful living.

In conclusion, mindfulness is a path to a richer, more meaningful experience of life, that grows only more vibrant with age. It is indeed an aging companion that brings tranquility, vigor, and a joyful zest for life. Dive into mindfulness; it's never too early to start.

Remember, mindful living isn't a destination, but a voyage, an intense, exhilarating journey towards a more fulfilled, serene, and vibrant self. And as you embark on this journey of 'Mindful Maturation,' remember that you're not just aging, but truly coming of age!

Chapter 4. Unlocking the Power of Acceptance

Acceptance is a powerful key, one that opens the door to a harmonious life. This beautiful state of mind transforms our interpretation of the world, alters our reactions and, therefore, builds a more serene and joyful experience. This state is not about ignoring the hardships and struggles that come with age; instead, it is about acknowledging them, learning from them, and cultivating a graceful journey.

4.1. The Essence of Acceptance

Acceptance is simply about giving yourself permission to experience your feelings without judgment. Whether it's about accepting physical changes, cognitive shifts, or altered lifestyle, acceptance helps you navigate these waters with an objective and empathetic approach. The essence of acceptance is in understanding that your age doesn't define you. It's not a state of stagnation; instead, it's another phase of life where you continue to grow and transform.

Remember, acceptance is not surrender; it's understanding. It does not rob you of your ability to make changes in your life. Instead, it equips you to respond to circumstances more effectively.

4.2. The Power of Mindful Acceptance

In the realm of mindful maturation, the practice of acceptance serves as a counteract to the stress of aging. As you maneuver the bumpy road of physical, emotional, and cognitive shifts, the tendency is to resist and fight these changes. However, pushing against the natural flow of life only elicits stress and discomfort.

On the other hand, mindful acceptance allows you to step back and observe your experiences without judgment, to lean into your feelings rather than avoid them. This helps in creating an empowering shift from avoidance to cognizance. Once you grasp this, you can manage your reactions better and carve out a more peaceful path for yourself.

4.3. Embracing Physical Changes

Reality dictates that our bodies mature over time, and the signs of aging will inevitably show. The wrinkles, the slower movements, the aching joints - they can be a source of distress if we judge ourselves based on the societal ideals of youth and vigor.

So, instead of struggling against these changes, why not embrace the reality with acceptance? Aches and pains might be an indication for you to slow down and adopt a gentler way of living. It's an opportunity to prioritize self-care, health-centric practices, and wholesome nutrition. Embrace these changes and make them your allies in the graceful aging journey.

4.4. Accepting Cognitive Shifts

The fear of cognitive decline is common, but remember not to equate aging with cognitive failure. It's an oversimplified notion that overshadows the real potential of the maturing mind. Yes, certain cognitive functions may slow down. However, this could be counteracted by a lifetime of accrued knowledge and insights.

With acceptance, you can break free from the negative paradigm and build a positive mindset about your cognitive abilities. It's a call to adopt habits that enhance cognitive health: mental stimulation, a balanced diet, regular exercise, and quality sleep. These, empowered by a mindful, accepting approach towards aging, can help maintain and boost cognitive health.

4.5. Altering Lifestyle with Grace

As the pace of life slows down, some activities you used to enjoy may become less accessible. However, acceptance can open up new windows of possibilities. Adopt new hobbies, explore different social activities, and learn new skills that fall within your capabilities. Aging doesn't mean retiring from an active lifestyle; it's about altering your approach and continuing the adventure in a more compassionate, enlightened tempo.

4.6. Letting Go of Invalidation

A part of acceptance is letting go of the desire for external validation. As we age, we can become more impressionable to what others think of our physical appearance or lifestyle. Acceptance nurtures independence from societal ideals and expectations, celebrating the unique journey that is yours. It encourages the authentic expression of self, unveiling the beauty of your individuality.

4.7. Journey to Acceptance

Begin your journey to acceptance by paying attention to your emotions. Identify any resistance, fear, or negativity you may have about aging, follow through these feelings. Ask yourself what's causing them? In answering this query, you clarify the hurdles that block your road to acceptance.

The practice of mindfulness is potent in this regard. With mindfulness, you cultivate self-awareness. You make room for tolerance and understanding, replacing the negative aspects of your existence with positivity. Mindfully accept what is and watch your perspective of life transform, one conscious breath at a time.

4.8. Conclusion

Unlocking the power of acceptance is not an overnight achievement. It calls for patience, understanding, and continuous effort. Be gentle with yourself through the process. Remember, this is your journey. Embrace the path of graceful aging with the invaluable key of acceptance. Every wrinkle, every gray hair, every laugh line - they are the badges of a life well-lived, a testament to your resilience and wisdom. Relish them, for they are part of the person you've become, unique and beautiful in your way. With acceptance, every step taken on this path becomes a dance, every breath is a music, and life becomes a grand, elegant ball.

Aging isn't a curse to be feared; it is a natural, beautiful process to be experienced. It is the greatest form of wisdom to practice acceptance in life, especially as one matures. In the orchestra of life, your music is essential, and so is every note you play - whether it's filled with youth or the wisdom of age. Embrace this mindfulness, and you'll find that the music of your life gets even richer with time.

Chapter 5. Healthy Habits for Graceful Aging

Aging is a natural process that every individual must embark upon at some point in their lives. Embarking on this journey with a healthy mind and body is imperative. In this context, we introduce you to a range of essential habits that promise to aid your voyage towards graceful aging.

5.1. Understanding the Importance of Regular Physical Activity

Physical activity is the key that unlocks a world of health benefits. It can boost your mood, keep your weight under control, and reduce the risks of numerous diseases.

Ensure that your day is generously sprinkled with physical movement. Choose activities that you enjoy so they can easily become part of your daily routine. Whether it's brisk walking, yoga, dancing, cycling, or swimming, the goal is to keep your body moving. Remember, it's never too late to start exercising.

5.2. Balanced Diet for Nutrient-Rich Living

As we age, the body's metabolism begins to slow down. Hence, incorporating a balanced diet rich in proteins, carbohydrates, vitamins, and minerals is indispensable.

Ensure that you consume plenty of fruits, vegetables, lean meats, dairy products, and whole grains. Cut down on processed foods, refined sugars, and unhealthy fats. Hydrate diligently and pay attention to portion control. A well-judged diet works wonders in keeping age-related ailments at bay.

5.3. Role of Regular Health Screenings and Check-ups

Preventive healthcare plays an indispensable role in the aging process. Regular health screenings and check-ups ensure that potential health issues are spotted and treated early.

Keep your vaccines up to date, and schedule regular appointments with your doctor. Routine monitoring of blood pressure, cholesterol levels, glucose levels, and bone density measurements can give you a clear picture of your overall health status.

5.4. Importance of Mental and Emotional Health

Mental and emotional wellbeing are as important as physical health. Keep your mind engaged with puzzles, books, and meaningful hobbies. Engage in social activities to nurture your friendships and relationships.

Mindfulness, meditation, and deep-breathing exercises can help you achieve inner peace and reduce stress. Pursuing a hobby, learning a new skill, or volunteering can provide a sense of purpose and spotlight the joy of living.

5.5. Prioritizing Sound Sleep

Quality sleep is often overlooked as a health pillar. However, it plays a significant role in maintaining optimal health and well-being.

Establish a calm and peaceful bedtime routine. Create a sleep-friendly environment that's dark, quiet, and cool. Avoid stimulants like caffeine and electronics close to bedtime. If you face persistent sleep issues, consult your doctor.

5.6. Daily Skincare Regime

Your skin experiences significant changes as you age. Keep it hydrated and nourished by following a daily skincare regime.

Moisturize daily, use sunscreen, and reduce exposure to the sun. Smoking can harm your skin, so it's better to quit. A healthy skin regime will not only make you feel good but also boost your overall self-esteem and confidence.

5.7. Understanding Your Body and Accepting Change

Aging can trigger changes in your body and life in general. Accepting these gracefully is key to mindful maturation.

It's important to listen to your body. Be aware of what it's telling you. Acknowledge its capabilities and limitations. Most importantly, remember, everyone ages at their own pace. Your journey is unique to you. Cherish it!

By incorporating these habits into your lifestyle, you're setting the stage for an ageless adventure. Embrace these habits and watch how beautifully life unfolds as you age. Remember, this journey is not about fighting aging. It's about acceptance and celebration. And it starts today! So, let's raise a toast to the grace and wisdom that comes with aging. Here's to a lifestyle and mindset shift towards mindful maturation!

Chapter 6. Refresh Your Perspective: Seeing Life Anew

Imagine holding up a prism to the sunlight; the rays of light refract, revealing a multitude of colors — a stunning, beautiful spectrum that always existed but needed just the right lens to be seen. Now, envision your life as this infinite beam of light and yourself holding the prism: the capacity to refract and reveal new colors — perspectives — that can transform your outlook on the world and your place within it. Welcome to a refreshing perspective: seeing your life anew.

6.1. The Importance of Perspective

The significance of perspective lies not just in its definition, but in the way it shapes our worldview. Your perspective is essentially your personal interpretation — the lens through which you view your experiences. Most of the time, these perspectives are so deeply ingrained; we're not even aware that we're wearing them.

With age comes the wisdom to recognize that we are more than our perspectives. Yet our viewpoints often limit us, for they are shaped by our past experiences — schooling, family, friendships, jobs, successes, failures and more. When you consciously step back and examine your perspectives, you're given a golden opportunity: to see life anew, through a lens that has been consciously chosen.

Let's take an example. Imagine viewing your life as a glass-half-empty because of the negative happenings your journey to maturation entails, such as health issues or societal bias about aging. But then, pause and think: what about the wealth of experience, the wisdom gained, the increased free time, and the ability to focus on personal growth and wellness? Suddenly, in the light of these considerations, that glass doesn't look quite so empty anymore — a shift in perspective.

6.2. Practicing Perspective-Reframing

We've established that perspective matters. The question, of course, is how do we begin to reframe our existing viewpoints? This is where mindfulness becomes instrumental. It allows us to become aware of our thought processes — to notice without judgment. Only when we know what's going on in our minds can we begin to change it.

One way to practice perspective-reframing is through mindful observation. Take five minutes each day to observe your surroundings: the smell of fresh coffee, the sound of birds chirping, the feel of your breath entering and exiting your body. As simple as it sounds, this momentary shift of focus from your inner thoughts to the outer world changes your wiring over time, enabling you to be more present and observant.

Another way is to make use of affirmations. An affirmation is a positive statement about yourself or your circumstances. For example, instead of saying "I'm too old", say with conviction, "I'm experienced and wise". Such self-talk shifts your perspective, breaking entrenched negative patterns and replacing them with positive ones. Remember, mindfulness and conscious action help us replace worn-out narratives.

6.3. Shifting Perception Through Compassionate Self-Talk

A powerful catalyst for perspective shifting is compassionate self-talk. Often, we're far harsher on ourselves than we would ever dream of being on others. This harshness creates a downward spiral of negative self-perception. Have you ever replayed a situation over and over, each time beating yourself up a bit more? It's destructive and, worse, unnecessary.

Compassionate self-talk helps break this cycle, allowing us to deal with ourselves as caring friends would. Here's how you can practice: next time you make a mistake, instead of indulging in self-directed negativity, say to yourself, "It's okay, everyone makes mistakes". Compassion towards oneself fosters a positive perspective, making us feel validated, nurtured, and, in turn, happy.

Remember, it's a process. Forgive yourself when you slip into old patterns, then firmly, gently, steer yourself back.

6.4. The Joy of A New Perspective

Bringing about a shift in your perspective is much like cultivating a garden. It requires patience, effort, and, above all, trust in the process. And the reward is well worth it. The ability to view life anew adds a wealth of richness to our everyday experiences. It enables us to derive joy from the simplest things and to weather storms with resilience and optimism.

When you start seeing life with a refreshed perspective, every sunrise feels different, every conversation feels different. You might find yourself enjoying the smallest of things - the laughter of a child, the aroma of baking bread, or the beauty of a blooming flower. Suddenly, life is full of a million new experiences waiting to be discovered.

Whatever age we might be, it's never too late to gain a new perspective on life. What's essential is the courage to question the status quo and the determination to effect change. After all, we are beings capable of growth, no matter the stage of life. You have the power right now to refract your light and reveal the stunning array of colors hidden within. The prism is in your hands.

Chapter 7. Wisdom in Wrinkles: Celebrating Age

There's no denying the physical transformations aging brings about. Wrinkles multiply, hair grows greyer, and the body moves at a slower pace than before. However, these changes have been ill-comprehended for many years. It's high time society re-evaluates its definition of aging and especially the beauty of wrinkles. Wrinkles represent countless smiles, hard-fought battles, and a life beautifully lived. They are the badges of honor that life bestows upon us.

7.1. Embracing the Aesthetic of Age

Have you ever paused to look at an old gnarled tree, its branches twisted and contorted with age? If you really take a moment to observe it, you'll notice its unique beauty. Every curve, every bumpy texture in the bark narrates a story. Like the old tree, wrinkles too tell a story – a story of how you have lived, of moments of joy, laughter, and sorrow. Aging, like the cycles of nature, is merely another phase of life that needs to be embraced as a part of our existence, instead of being shunned out of fear. Aging, in itself, is a beautiful process if we find the grace to see it for what it truly is.

7.2. Wrinkles: The Unseen Layers

Beyond their exterior form, wrinkles symbolize life's unseen layers - the triumphs and tribulations, the lessons learned, and the wisdom earned. Each wrinkle is a testament to an experience lived—whether it be a triumphant victory, a disastrous failure, or an unexpected revelation. We all carry these stories with us, etched into the very lines of our faces, a silent whisper of our personal histories.

Aging doesn't mean an end to experiences, either. Instead, aging paves the way for new experiences and fresh insights into life. As we move on from one chapter of life to another, we find the deep crevices of experience making us more robust and wise. We should not avoid the mirror for fear of seeing our age. We should look proudly at those laugh lines, crow's feet, and furrowed brows, knowing that they're evidence of a life well-lived.

7.3. The Beauty of Aging Mindfully

Aging mindfully is all about recognizing and embracing every change that comes our way. It involves acknowledging the physical changes and adapting our minds to accept and cherish these transformations. Mindful aging calls us to fully inhabit our aging bodies, to live life with all its vicissitudes with grace and gratitude. It is about connecting with the wisdom within and beyond our wrinkled exterior, about finding joy, love, and contentment in life's every phase.

7.4. Aging and Wisdom: An Inextricable Bond

Life has a generous way of dealing lessons in the guise of experiences. Each passing moment is a chance to grow and evolve, and aging brings a unique perspective to this universal truth. It's quite magical how our minds mature as we age. We not only become more resilient but also more empathetic, understanding the world and its ways from a broader, seasoned perspective. Our wrinkles embody this wisdom, serving as daily reminders of the lessons we've learned over our lifetime.

7.5. A Harmonious Association with Time

One of the greatest benefits of aging is the relationship we develop with time. When we're young, we often view time as an infinite resource. But as we age wisely, we realize that time isn't limitless. This comprehension makes us value the present – the "now" – even more.

When you come to terms with your finite timeline, you consciously prioritize what's truly important: Happiness, peace, companionship, health, and sometimes, looking back to cherish the beautiful life you've lived so far. Recognizing the delicate beauty of transience helps us live more meaningful lives.

7.6. Celebrating Your Age

Every new wrinkle, every grey hair, every memory etched into your heart is a reason to celebrate. Each passing year offers a higher vantage point from where you can look back at the winding road of your journey so far and smile at the beautiful tapestry you've woven. There's a unique beauty in standing tall with grace, living each day in the rainbow of emotions life offers, and loving the person you see in the mirror, made so uniquely beautiful and wise by the passing years.

Celebrate your age, not as a countdown but as a count-up. Count all your blessings, all those beautiful moments, all those life lessons learned, all the love you've given and received, and all the wisdom you've gained. "Mindful Maturation: Graceful Aging for Baby Boomers" is not just about accepting aging but about rejoicing in its wisdom and absolute beauty. To age is to have lived - and to have lived is the real accomplishment.

Chapter 8. The Baby Boomer's Guide to Mental Fitness

Mental fitness, like physical fitness, needs constant nurturing. Unpacking its many facets, we aim to provide Baby Boomers with a comprehensive guide to keeping their minds sharp, open, and invigorated.

8.1. Understanding Mental Fitness

Mental fitness refers to our cognitive and emotional wellbeing. It's not just about memory, but a complex web of psychological flexibility, emotional regulation, creativity, and resilience. In essence, mental fitness is the gym membership for the mind you never knew you needed. It's the exercise regime that keeps neurons vibrant and emotions balanced.

8.2. The Power of Mindfulness

Mindfulness is not a lofty concept held by monks in remote monasteries. It's a practical tool for daily life. Mindfulness helps us to live fully in the present moment, rooting the mind into the 'now' and training it to quieten the chatter of the past and the future.

An easy start to mindfulness is mindful breathing. All it requires is awareness of the breath. Sit comfortably, close your eyes, and focus on your breathing. Notice the rhythm, the rise and fall of your chest, the sensation of breath entering and leaving your body. Whenever your mind wanders, gently bring it back to observing your breath.

8.3. Cognitive Stimulation: Keep the Neurons Dashing

Cognitive stimulation activities help in keeping the mind active and agile. These could include memory games, puzzles, or learning new skills.

Exploring a new language can be a great cognitive exercise, challenging the mind to form new neural connections. Similarly, picking up a musical instrument dusted in the attic can also be beneficial.

Strive for mental agility, not perfection. The objective is to initiate the process of learning, stretching the boundaries of comfort, and shaking off mental inertia.

8.4. Physical Activity: Embrace Movement

An essential yet often overlooked aspect of mental health is regular physical activity. It boosts mood and sleep quality, reduces stress, and increases overall cognitive performance.

Regular physical activity does not necessarily mean strenuous exercise. It can be as simple as taking a brisk walk, gardening, or practising yoga. The key is to find an activity you love and make it a routine.

8.5. Connections: Harness the Power of Relationships

Our mental health and well-being are significantly influenced by our relationships. Staying connected with family, friends, and community helps us feel valued, understood, and emotionally fulfilled.

Seek ways to cultivate and sustain meaningful relationships. Engage in community activities, meet friends regularly, and explore online platforms to connect with people sharing similar interests.

8.6. Nutritional Gains: Feed Your Brain

Your brain needs the right nutrients to function correctly, just like any other organ. Omega-3 fatty acids, antioxidants, B-vitamins, and proteins are essential in maintaining a healthy brain.

Enhance your diet with a variety of fruits, vegetables, lean protein, and sources of healthy fats, such as avocadoes, walnuts, or chia seeds. Also, drink plenty of water and reduce the consumption of processed foods, sugar, and caffeine.

8.7. Embrace Positivity: The Catalyst of Wellness

Adopting a positive outlook is not about denying the realities of life. It's about coping wisely. It's about uplifting yourself despite the hurtles, seeing them as lessons rather than failures.

A gratitude journal can help foster positivity. Before going to bed, jot down three things you were grateful for during the day. This simple act gradually rewires the brain to focus more on positivity, helping us feel happier and more content.

8.8. The Beauty of Sleep

Sleep is vital for cognitive function. It replenishes the mind and body, clears out brain toxins, and solidifies memory.

Prioritizing sleep helps in mood regulation, memory consolidation, and overall mental fitness. Try to maintain regular sleep schedules, create a calm and dark bedroom environment, and limit exposure to blue light before sleeping.

8.9. Stress Management: Respect Your Limits

Stress management doesn't necessarily mean living a life devoid of stress, but learning to manage reaction to stressful situations.

Mindfulness, positive coping mechanisms, and physical activity are effective stress busters. Sometimes, it also means saying no and setting boundaries, respecting your physical and emotional limits.

It's essential to remember that mental maturation is a journey, not a destination. It is the unfolding process of growing wiser, becoming more compassionate to oneself, and carving a life that radiates deep contentment and joy. It's not a distinct chapter of life but an ongoing narrative, an enchantingly vibrant tapestry woven through the threads of experiences, wisdom, mistakes, and growth.

Chapter 9. Cultivating Positive Relationships

We possess dual existence as individuals isolated within ourselves and as creatures of society, engaged in constant interplay with the people around us. Genuine and positive relationships, undeniably, lay the foundation of an enlightened and enriching life, fulfilling in equal measures for the baby boomer generation as well as those in the prime of their youth. Journey into the incredible world of harmonious connections as we delve deeper into this chapter.

9.1. The Importance of Positive Relationships

Relationships rule our social sphere, weaving a closely-knit fabric of collective consciousness throughout our lives. From the immediate family to extended kinship, friendships, and romantic partnerships, relationships mold our experiences, influence our perspectives, shape our behaviors, and contribute significantly to our overall wellbeing. For baby boomers stepping into the golden chapter of their lives, maintaining potent, positive relationships becomes more critical than ever. They serve as a conduit of emotional support, intellectual stimulation, a reassuring buffer against loneliness and isolation, and an invigorating trigger for happiness and contentment.

9.2. Nurturing Relationships: A Mindful Approach

Nurturing relationships is like cultivating a garden, requiring dedication, patience, and mindful efforts. As we age, our physical energy may reduce, but our emotional intelligence certainly ascends. This ability to empathize, understand, and handle emotions effectively is the secret ingredient in the recipe for durable, enriching relationships.

Always remember, communication is king. Frequent and mindful exchanges foster understanding and sustain the vitality of your relationships. Be it sharing jovial anecdotes from the past or discussing an enlightening book you recently read, strive to keep the communication lively, genuine, and frequent.

9.3. The Role of Compassionate Understanding

Understanding flows mellifluously from the reservoir of compassion. Small gestures of kindness echoing genuine care and concern for our loved ones can significantly reinforce the bonds we share. Take a moment each day to comprehend the thoughts, feelings, and experiences your loved ones are grappling with. This compassionate vantage point will unveil perspectives unthought of, creating a bridge of emotional intimacy and trust.

9.4. Embracing Forgiveness

Over the course of our shared lives, misunderstandings, misconceptions, and disputes are inevasible. Let forgiveness flourish in the garden of your relationships, cultivating an environment of growth and mutual acceptance. Forgiving is not forgetting; it is the conscious choice of focusing on the positive notwithstanding past hurt. It frees our hearts of resentment and absorbs the soothing elixir of compassion, enriching the relationship.

9.5. Setting Healthy Boundaries

Knowing when to step forward and when to draw back is crucial. Constructive boundaries embody respect and understanding. They reflect that we not only respect our privacy and personal space but also that of others. This reciprocal approach ensures the longevity of relationships and safeguards us from exhaustion or unfair impositions.

It's not the quantity; it's the strength and depth of your relationships that truly count. A handful of deeply nourishing relationships can weave a deeply fulfilling life than a crowd of superficial acquaintances. This is the soulful symphony of positive connections. As we strike the right balance of love, understanding, communication, and empathy, we transcend the ordinary boundaries of association and embark on a delightful journey of synergism.

In conclusion, don't view the realm of relationships as a cumbersome task, but as a joyful journey. With each forged connection, you piece together the jigsaw puzzle of humanity. Dive into the vibrant canvas of human interactions, and paint your narrative with vibrant colors of compassion, understanding, joy, and life. And remember, while these guidelines are here to lead you, the relationships you choose to cultivate and how you go about doing so, is ultimately, uniquely yours. Listen to your heart and allow it to navigate your path. Embrace the beauty of your journey as you gracefully stride into the golden epoch of life, hand in hand with your loved ones.

Chapter 10. Rediscover the Joys of Learning

Aging invites a renewed impetus to explore and learn. Knowledge, as they say, has no retirement age, it is a lifelong journey of discovery. Understanding this, you begin to comprehend the immense joy and satisfaction learning can offer even at the precipice of your life's Winter. Here, we guide you through the labyrinth of learning in the later stages of life.

10.1. Building a Learning Mindset

An imperative step towards rekindling the thrill of learning is to build a positive learning mindset. It's not uncommon for the elderly to apprehend learning new skills or refreshing old ones due to barriers like fear of failure, outdated beliefs about learning, or the misconception that learning decreases with age.

But, as recent neuroscientific research reveals, the human mind, regardless of age, possesses an astonishing capacity to adapt, learn, and grow—a concept known as neuroplasticity. So, devoid of all inhibitions, embrace the wisdom of being a lifelong learner.

Step into the learner's shoes with enthusiasm and grace, remembering that each new idea learned or each skill honed brings you closer to personal expansion. This mindset of growth allows you to embrace challenges, persist against obstacles, see effort as a path to mastery, learn from criticism, and find lessons and inspiration from others' success.

10.2. Circles of Learning

Effective learning in later life often thrives in interactive, social environments. Consider engaging in collaborative learning circles with other eager learners. Together, you can explore a variety of subjects, from literature to art, science to history, or perhaps a language you've always desired to learn.

These groups provide encouragement and a sense of camaraderie, reinvigorating your passion for knowledge. Additionally, the use of discussion and debate enriches critical thinking and promotes a deeper understanding of the topics at hand, mirroring the adage that we learn best when we learn together.

10.3. Exploit the Digital Age

The digital age, filled with online courses and educational platforms, makes learning accessible for everyone, anytime, anywhere. Use technology as a tool to expand your mental horizons. Online learning platforms like Coursera, Khan Academy, Udemy, and others offer a myriad of courses across multiple disciplines, often for free or for a modest fee.

Don't let technology intimidate you. Instead, choose to see it as a pathway, a directory full of all the world's knowledge, ready for you to delve in and explore.

10.4. Celebrate Each Victory

One pivotal concept to instill in your learning journey is to celebrate every little progress made. When you learn something new, acknowledge it, and take a moment to relish the victory. It's not just about reaching the end goal, but about embracing the entire journey. Every moment of understanding, every increment of knowledge gained, and every challenge overcome is a reason to celebrate.

10.5. Art of Mindful Learning

Lastly, but most crucially, practice mindful learning. Be present in each moment of the learning process. Pay attention to the information, the textures of your comprehension, and the emotions that come along. Mindful learning not only optimizes memory and focus but also lights the path with the gentle glow of consciousness, adding a richer texture to your learning journey.

Embarking on this voyage of rediscovery, every nuance of knowledge brightened by the soft, wise embers of experience, you let go of the urgency, the rush, and simply enjoy. Enjoy the learning for learning's sake, wrapped in the warm embrace of age's quiet wisdom.

For some, the older years may represent a time of diminishing, of closing down, or of loss. Yet, your journey demonstrates conclusively that these years can be a time of the most tremendous growth and expansion. Realign your course with learning, keep your mind as agile as your spirit, and you will discover the golden years of life aren't the end of the rainbow but rather, a brand new, glorious chapter, brimming with possibilities and joy.

Dive into this chapter of learning with an open heart, a curious mind, and a daring spirit, and you'll find it's as enchanting, as engaging - if not more so, as those first days of school, where the world unfolded before you in the pages of your textbooks.

Keep learning, keep growing and thrive in the sweet cadence of enriching wisdom. Each new day is another opportunity for discovery. Keep that flame of curiosity alive and burning bright. After all, life, in all its miraculous phases, is a grand voyage of learning.

Embrace the delightful art of continuous learning and remember: it's never too late to learn and never too old to discover the joys of gaining knowledge; because you are still growing, still evolving, and as long as you live, there's so much more to learn, and so much more to become.

Chapter 11. Creating a Legacy: Your Contribution to the World

The human being is a complex amalgamation of experiences, insights, knowledge, and value. As we navigate the path of life, we invariably leave our mark on the world in countless components, big and small. The essence of 'creating a legacy' lies precisely in acknowledging this footprint and expanding it consciously into something meaningful, impactful, and long-lasting, that outlives our immediate physical existence.

11.1. Understanding your Legacy

Your legacy is the valuable imprint you leave behind for future generations. It's your contribution to the world, a testament of your life, a measure of the influence you've had on people, places, and issues during your journey on earth. Your legacy is subjective to your personal ideals, values, experiences, and aspirations. For some, it could be as intimate as raising well-rounded children, while others might aspire to impact society on a larger scale through philanthropic efforts or revolutionary ideas.

Delve into introspection. Ponder over your life. What do you count among your most significant accomplishments? Which moments filled your heart with the glow of satisfaction? Above all, what satisfaction would you derive from the world you leave behind?

11.2. Guidepost to Defining your Legacy

Begin by reflecting on what matters to you the most. What values do you hold dear? What have been your passions, or what inspires strong emotions in you?

Synthesize this understanding into a concrete idea. A clear notion gives you a solid platform to construct your legacy. It could be commitment to social work, fostering education, environmental conservation, or technological innovation.

Next, reflect on your skills and resources. What are you best equipped to contribute? Your legacy must harness your capabilities. Your skillset and resources play a crucial part in effectuating your legacy.

11.3. Crafting your Vision

Once you've explored your values and capabilities, the next step is to envision your legacy. This vision essentially paints a picture of the world you'd like to contribute towards.

Begin by visualizing the broader picture—your ultimate aspiration. Keeping that as your guiding light, establish a distinct mission that underlines your purpose and outlines the path to realize your vision.

To streamline your efforts and maintain focus, set clear, measurable goals. These should focus on the impact you desire to make. Remember, however grand or humble, your vision should resonate with your core values and align with your capabilities.

11.4. Taking Incremental Steps

Your legacy unfolds as you progress through life, and so, it calls for consistent efforts over time. Start small, leveraging everyday opportunities to impact your surroundings positively. These small steps contribute to the larger picture and set an example for the people looking up to you.

Kindling a child's curiosity, lending a listening ear to a friend, or planting a tree might seem trivial, but they are indeed powerful gestures that influence the world in their own right. These are small building blocks nurturing a legacy of compassion, understanding, and sustainability.

11.5. Balancing Advancement with Service

Many associate leaving a legacy with acquiring financial or social success. Yes, accumulating resources can provide a stepping stone towards creating a more expansive legacy. However, the essence of legacy isn't simply about the heights to which you rise, but how you enable others to rise along with you, rooting deep in the balance between personal advancement and communal service.

Aspiring to excel and accumulate resources is not contradictory to serving your community. Instead, they can foster each other in a synergistic manner. Success can often create opportunities to make a difference and vice versa.

11.6. Teach to Empower

Embracing the role of a mentor can establish a lasting legacy. The wisdom and experiences you share can empower others to enhance their life trajectory, fostering a legacy that thrives through generations.

Teaching isn't limited to formal education. Every interaction provides an opportunity to learn and teach. By sharing your wisdom and nurturing others' growth, you sow the seeds of your legacy in their hearts.

11.7. Conclusion: Stay True to You

Embarking on the voyage of 'creating a legacy', remember that your desire to leave an impact must be intertwined with your unique self. It shouldn't be driven by social expectations or a pursuit of validation, but a profound aspiration to contribute. Your legacy is an extension of who you are, who you aspire to be, and the world you wish to co-create. You leave a legacy by living a life that's authentic to you and meaningful for others.

By following the steps delineated in this chapter, you can create a legacy imbued with your wisdom, values, and unique insights that echo into the future. We hope it presents a gentle nudge propelling you to consider, cultivate, and cherish your contribution to the world. Even as you continue your journey of mindful maturation, remember - through your legacy, you etch indelible prints on the sands of time.